WEIGHT LOSS DIET FOR BEGINNERS

The Complete Guide to Losing Pounds and Changing Your Life

DR. JOSEPHINE W. PACK

TABLE OF CONTENTS

DELICIOUS RECIPE

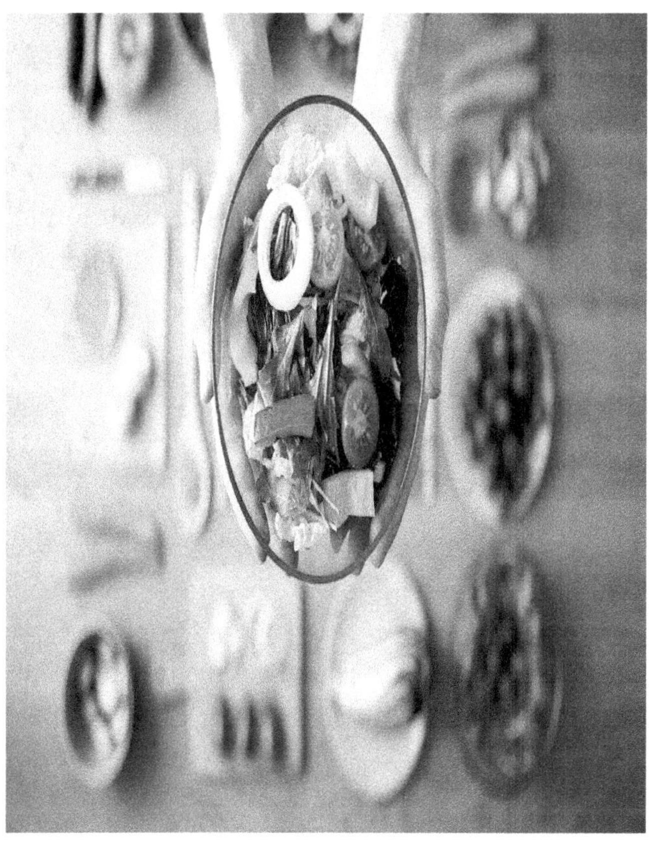

INTRODUCTION

Mrs. Smith had always wished to lose those obstinate pounds that refused to leave her body no matter what she did. Mrs. Smith was frustrated and dejected until she came across this extraordinary book named "Weight Loss Diet for Beginners" that offered a novel strategy to attain her objectives.

Mrs. Smith quickly scanned through the pages of the book, uncovering a wealth of information and useful recommendations. The book's author, Dr. Pack, is a famous nutritionist who emphasizes the significance of a holistic approach to weight management that includes a good diet, regular exercise, and a positive outlook.

Mrs. Smith set off on her weight reduction quest with renewed zeal after hearing Dr. Pack's encouraging comments. She emptied her cabinet of processed foods and replaced them with fresh fruits, veggies, and lean meats. She used this book to prepare tasty but healthy meals that pleased her appetites while also nourishing her body. Physical exercise is also important. Mrs. Smith began with easy workouts, gradually building stamina and strength. She found the pleasure of movement, whether it was a leisurely stroll around the park or a joyful dance lesson.

Days became weeks, and weeks become months. Mrs. Smith observed that her clothing were fitting looser, her energy levels were increasing, and her confidence was rising. This book had been her constant friend, guiding and supporting her every step of the journey. Mrs. Smith stood proudly in front of the mirror, marveling at her metamorphosis as time passed. The pounds vanished, and she exuded a renewed feeling of vibrancy and self-assurance. "Weight Loss Diet for Beginners" had been her guiding light, enabling her to attain her objectives in a shockingly short amount of time. Mrs. Smith decided to share her success story with others, spreading the word about the transformational power of this book that had permanently transformed her life.

CHAPTER 1. Salad Mediterranean

Ingredients:

Salad with mixed greens, cherry tomatoes, cucumbers, olives, feta cheese, lemon juice, olive oil, salt, and pepper.

Preparation:

Toss all of the ingredients in a bowl and season with lemon juice, olive oil, salt, and pepper.

Stuffed Bell Peppers with Quinoa

Ingredients:

Bell peppers, cooked quinoa, black beans, maize, chopped tomatoes, onion, garlic, cumin, chili powder, salt, and pepper are among the ingredients.

Preparation:

Sauté the onion and garlic in a pan until tender. Combine the black beans, corn, chopped tomatoes, cumin, chili powder, salt, and pepper in a mixing bowl. Incorporate the cooked quinoa. Bake for

25-30 minutes, stuffing the bell peppers with the mixture.

Steamed Broccoli with Grilled Chicken Breast

Ingredients:
Chicken breast, lemon juice, garlic powder, salt, pepper, and broccoli are the ingredients.

Preparation:
Season the chicken breast with lemon juice, garlic powder, salt, and pepper before cooking. Broccoli should be steamed until soft. Grilled chicken breast should be served with steamed broccoli.

Omelet with Spinach and Mushrooms

Ingredients:
Eggs, spinach, mushrooms, onion, salt, pepper, and olive oil are among the ingredients.

Preparation:
Sauté the onion and mushrooms until softened. Cook until the spinach has wilted. Separately, season

the eggs with salt and pepper. Cook, stirring occasionally, until the eggs are set and the bottom is golden. Cook for another minute after flipping the omelet. Serve immediately.

Lentil Soup

Ingredients:
lentils, onion, carrots, celery, garlic, vegetable broth, cumin, paprika, salt, and pepper.

Preparation:
Saute the onion, carrots, celery, and garlic in a large saucepan until softened. Combine the lentils, vegetable broth, cumin, paprika, salt, and pepper in a mixing bowl. Serve immediately.

CHAPTER 2. Lettuce Wraps with Tuna Salad

Ingredients:

Canned tuna, Greek yogurt, lemon juice, Dijon mustard, celery, red onion, salt, pepper, and lettuce leaves are the ingredients.

Preparation:

Combine the canned tuna, Greek yogurt, lemon juice, Dijon mustard, celery, red onion, salt, and pepper in a mixing dish. Wrap the lettuce leaves in lettuce leaves with the tuna salad. Chill before serving.

Noodles with Zucchini and Tomato Sauce

Ingredients:

Zucchini, tomato sauce, garlic, olive oil, basil, salt, and pepper are the main ingredients.

Preparation:

Spiralize the zucchini to make noodles. Cook until the garlic is aromatic. Sauté the zucchini noodles for a few minutes, or until soft. Heat the tomato sauce in a saucepan. Add basil, salt, and pepper to taste. Serve immediately.

Salmon Baked with Asparagus

Ingredients:
Salmon filets, lemon juice, garlic, salt, pepper, asparagus spears, and olive oil are the ingredients.

Preparation:
Place the salmon filets on a baking pan and set aside. Squeeze fresh lemon juice over the fish and season with salt and pepper. Arrange the spears of asparagus around the fish. Season the asparagus with salt and pepper and drizzle with olive oil. Bake for 12-15 minutes, or until the salmon is well cooked and the asparagus is soft.

Fried Cauliflower Rice

Ingredients:
Cauliflower, carrots, peas, onion, garlic, soy sauce, sesame oil, eggs, and green onions are among the ingredients.

Preparation:
Prepare the cauliflower by cutting it into florets and pulsing it in a food processor until it resembles rice

grains. Cook the carrots, peas, onion, and garlic in a large pan until softened. Place the veggies on one side of the pan and the eggs on the other. Scramble the eggs, then combine them with the veggies. Stir-fry the cauliflower rice for a few minutes in the skillet. Drizzle with sesame oil and soy sauce. Garnish with green onions, if desired.

Salad with Greek Chicken

Ingredients:
Grilled chicken breast, mixed greens, cucumber, cherry tomatoes, red onion, Kalamata olives, feta cheese, lemon juice, olive oil, salt, and pepper are among the ingredients.

Preparation:
Thinly slice the grilled chicken breast. Combine mixed greens, sliced cucumber, cherry tomatoes, red onion, Kalamata olives, and feta cheese in a large mixing basin. Top with the cut chicken. Toss thoroughly before serving.

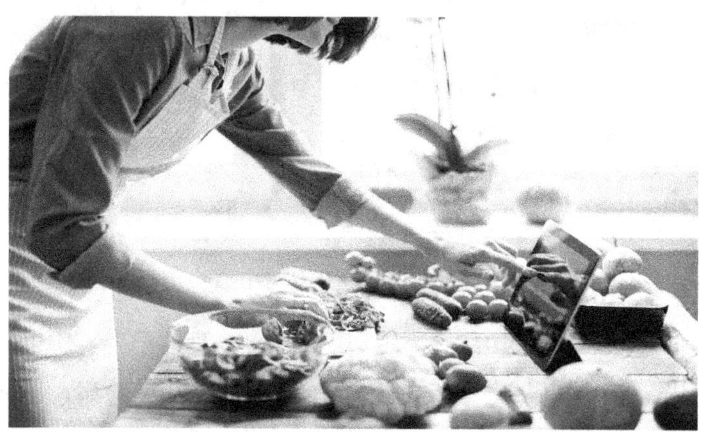

Ingredients:

Sweet potatoes, black beans, chopped tomatoes, onion, garlic, chili powder, cumin, paprika, vegetable broth, salt, and pepper are among the ingredients.

Preparation:

Saute the onion and garlic in a large saucepan until tender. Cook for a few minutes after adding the cubed sweet potatoes. Combine the black beans, chopped tomatoes, chili powder, cumin, paprika, salt, and pepper in a mixing bowl. Bring the vegetable broth to a boil in a saucepan. Reduce the heat to low and cook for 20-25 minutes, or until the sweet potatoes are cooked. Serve immediately.

Veggie Stir-Fry

Ingredients:
Broccoli, bell peppers, carrots, snap peas, and mushrooms, garlic, ginger, soy sauce, and sesame oil.

Preparation:
Cut the veggies into bite-sized pieces before starting. Heat sesame oil in a wok or big pan over high heat. Stir in the veggies until crisp-tender. Toss the veggies in the soy sauce to coat. Serve immediately.

Omelet with Egg Whites, Spinach, and Feta

Ingredients:
Egg whites, spinach, feta cheese, onion, salt, and pepper are the main ingredients.

Preparation:

In a mixing dish, whisk together the egg whites, salt, and pepper. Sauté the onion in a pan until transparent. Cook until the spinach has wilted. Cook until the egg whites have set in the skillet. Fold the omelet in half and top with feta cheese. Cook for 1 minute more, until the cheese has melted. Serve immediately.

Smoothie with Berries and Protein

Ingredients:

Unsweetened almond milk, protein powder, spinach, chia seeds, and honey (optional).

Preparation:

Blend together mixed berries, almond milk, protein powder, spinach, chia seeds, and honey (if using) in a blender. If necessary, adjust the consistency by adding additional almond milk.

Stir-Fry with Shrimp and Vegetables

Ingredients:

Shrimp, broccoli, bell peppers, snow peas, carrots, garlic, ginger, soy sauce, and sesame oil are among the ingredients.

Preparation:

Heat sesame oil in a wok or big pan over high heat. Stir-fry the veggies in the pan until crisp-tender. Pour the soy sauce over the shrimp in the pan. Cook for another minute after tossing everything together. Serve immediately.

CHAPTER 4. Berries with Almonds Greek Yogurt

Ingredients:
Greek yogurt, berries (strawberries, blueberries, raspberries), almonds, and honey (optional).

Preparation:
To begin, spoon Greek yogurt into a bowl. Garnish with berries and almonds. If desired, drizzle with honey. Before eating, combine everything.

Skewers of chicken and vegetables

Ingredients:
Chicken breast, bell peppers, red onion, zucchini, cherry tomatoes, olive oil, lemon juice, garlic, salt, and pepper are the ingredients.

Preparation:
Prepare the chicken breast by cutting it into bits. Thread the skewers with the chicken, bell peppers, red onion, zucchini, and cherry tomatoes. Combine the olive oil, lemon juice, minced garlic, salt, and

pepper in a mixing bowl. Brush the skewers with the marinade. Grill the skewers until the chicken and veggies are cooked through. Serve immediately.

Stir-Fry with Tofu and Vegetables

Ingredients:
Firm tofu, broccoli, mushrooms, snap peas, bell peppers, garlic, ginger, soy sauce, and sesame oil are among the ingredients.

Preparation:
To begin, cut the tofu into cubes. Heat sesame oil in a wok or big pan over high heat. Cook until the tofu is gently browned. Set the tofu aside after removing it from the pan. Stir-fry the veggies in the pan until crisp-tender. Pour the soy sauce over the tofu in the pan. Cook for another minute after tossing everything together. Serve immediately.

Lettuce Wraps with Turkey

Ingredients:
Lean ground turkey, lettuce leaves, mushrooms, water chestnuts, garlic, ginger, soy sauce, and sesame oil are the ingredients.

Preparation:

Cook the ground turkey in a pan until it is browned. Mix in the minced garlic and ginger, as well as the mushrooms and water chestnuts. Boil for a few minutes. Add the soy sauce and sesame oil. Combine all of the ingredients. Wrap the lettuce leaves in lettuce leaves with the turkey mixture. Chill before serving.

Parmesan-Roasted Brussels Sprouts

Ingredients:

Brussels sprouts, olive oil, garlic powder, Parmesan cheese, salt, and pepper are the ingredients.

Preparation:

Trim the Brussels sprouts' ends and chop them in half. Combine the Brussels sprouts, olive oil, garlic powder, salt, and pepper in a mixing bowl. Place them on a baking pan. Roast the Brussels sprouts for 25-30 minutes, or until crispy and golden.

Ingredients:

Lemon, fresh herbs (such as thyme, parsley, or dill), olive oil, salt, and pepper.

Preparation:

In a baking dish, place the fish filets. Fresh lemon juice should be squeezed over the fish. Fresh herbs, finely chopped, should be sprinkled over the fish. Bake the fish for 12-15 minutes, or until opaque and flaky with a fork. Serve immediately.

Pesto Zucchini with Carrot Noodles

Ingredients:

Zucchini, carrots, basil pesto, cherry tomatoes, pine nuts, and Parmesan cheese are among the ingredients.

Preparation:

Spiralize the zucchini and carrots to make noodles. Sauté the zucchini and carrot noodles for a few minutes, or until soft. Combine the basil pesto and cherry tomatoes in a mixing bowl. Cook until the tomatoes have softened somewhat. In a dry skillet, toast the pine nuts until brown. Toasted pine nuts and grated Parmesan cheese are sprinkled over the noodles. Serve hot.

Salad with Blackened Chicken

Ingredients:
Blackened chicken breast, mixed greens, cherry tomatoes, avocado, red onion, corn, black beans, lime juice, olive oil, salt, and pepper are the ingredients.

Preparation:
Prepare the blackened chicken breast by slicing it into thin pieces. Combine mixed greens, cherry tomatoes, sliced avocado, thinly sliced red onion, corn, and black beans in a large mixing dish. Season with lime juice, olive oil, salt, and pepper to taste. Top with the cut chicken. Toss thoroughly before serving.

Curry with Lentils and Vegetables

Ingredients:

Lentils, onion, bell peppers, cauliflower, carrots, garlic, ginger, curry powder, coconut milk, vegetable broth, salt, and pepper are among the ingredients.

Preparation:

Saute the onion, bell peppers, cauliflower, carrots, garlic, and ginger in a large saucepan until softened. Combine the lentils, curry powder, coconut milk, vegetable broth, salt, and pepper in a mixing bowl. Cook, stirring occasionally, for 20-25 minutes, or until the lentils and veggies are cooked. Serve immediately with rice or quinoa.

Parmesan Baked Eggplant

Ingredients:

Eggplant, marinara sauce, mozzarella cheese, Parmesan cheese, breadcrumbs, olive oil, salt, and pepper are the ingredients.

Preparation:

Make rounds with the eggplant. Sprinkle salt on both sides of the eggplant slices and let aside for 15 minutes to allow moisture to escape. Using paper towels, rinse and wipe dry. Each eggplant slice should be dipped in olive oil and then coated in breadcrumbs. Bake the breaded eggplant slices for 15-20 minutes, or until golden brown, on a baking pan. Remove the slices from the oven and sprinkle with marinara sauce, mozzarella cheese, and grated Parmesan cheese. Return to the oven for 10 minutes more, or until the cheese is melted and bubbling. Serve immediately.

Mexican Quinoa Salad

Ingredients:
Quinoa, black beans, maize, cherry tomatoes, avocado, red onion, cilantro, lime juice, olive oil, cumin, chili powder, salt, and pepper are the ingredients.

Preparation:
Combine cooked quinoa, black beans, corn, halved cherry tomatoes, diced avocado, finely chopped red onion, and cilantro in a large mixing bowl. Lime juice, olive oil, cumin, chili powder, salt, and pepper to taste. Toss everything together until everything is fully integrated. As a delightful Mexican-inspired quinoa dish, serve hot or chilled.

CHAPTER 6. Salmon Steamed with Lemon and Dill

Ingredients:

Salmon filets, lemon slices, fresh dill, salt, and pepper are the main ingredients.

Preparation:

Place the salmon filets in a steamer basket and set aside. Season with salt and pepper to taste. Garnish each filet with lemon slices and fresh dill sprigs. Steam the salmon for 10-12 minutes, or until it is cooked through and flakes readily with a fork.

Salad with Asian Cucumbers

Ingredients:

Cucumbers, rice vinegar, soy sauce, sesame oil, garlic, ginger, red pepper flakes, and sesame seeds are among the ingredients.

Preparation:

Prepare the cucumbers by slicing them thinly and placing them in a basin. Whisk together rice vinegar, soy sauce, sesame oil, chopped garlic, grated ginger, and a sprinkle of red pepper flakes in a separate bowl. To coat, pour the dressing over the cut cucumbers.

Turkey and Quinoa Stuffed Bell Peppers

Ingredients:
Bell peppers, ground turkey, cooked quinoa, onion, garlic, tomato sauce, Italian seasoning, salt, and pepper are among the ingredients.

Preparation:
Cook until the chopped onion and minced garlic are softened. Add cooked quinoa, tomato sauce, Italian seasoning, salt, and pepper to taste. Fill the bell peppers with the mixture and lay them on a baking tray. Bake for 25-30 minutes, or until the peppers are soft and the mixture is hot.

Smoothie with greens

Ingredients:
Spinach, kale, cucumber, green apple, lemon juice, ginger, water or coconut water, ice cubes

Preparation:

Blend spinach, kale, sliced cucumber, chopped green apple, lemon juice, grated ginger, water or coconut. If necessary, adjust the consistency by adding additional water.

Stir-Fry with Turkey and Vegetables

Ingredients:

Lean ground turkey, broccoli, snap peas, bell peppers, carrots, garlic, ginger, soy sauce, and sesame oil are among the ingredients.

Preparation:

Cook the ground turkey in a pan until it is browned. Broccoli florets, snap peas, sliced bell peppers, and shredded carrots are all good additions. Stir-fry the veggies until they are crisp-tender. Drizzle with sesame oil and soy sauce. Cook for another minute after tossing everything together. Serve immediately.

Stuffed Chicken Breast in Greek Style

Ingredients:

Chicken breast, spinach, feta cheese, sun-dried tomatoes, garlic, lemon juice, olive oil, salt, and pepper are the ingredients.

Preparation:

Butterfly the chicken breast by slicing it horizontally but not all the way through, creating a book-style opening. Season with salt and pepper on the interior. In a mixing bowl, combine chopped spinach, crumbled feta cheese, minced sun-dried tomatoes, minced garlic, lemon juice, and olive oil. Spoon the mixture over one side of the butterflied chicken breast and seal it with the other side. If required, secure with toothpicks. Spread the filled chicken breast out on a baking sheet and sprinkle with olive oil. Bake for 25-30 minutes, or until the chicken is well done. Before serving, remove the toothpicks.

CHAPTER 7. Stir-Fry Cauliflower Rice

Ingredients:

Cauliflower, other vegetables (including bell peppers, carrots, peas, and maize), garlic, ginger, soy sauce, and sesame oil are among the ingredients.

Preparation:

Prepare the cauliflower by cutting it into florets and pulsing it in a food processor until it resembles rice grains. Stir in the minced garlic and grated ginger for a minute, or until fragrant. Stir in the cauliflower rice for a few minutes, or until it softens. Place the cauliflower rice on one side of the pan and the veggies on the other. Cook until the veggies are crisp-tender. Combine everything and sprinkle with soy sauce. Stir-fry for another minute, or until everything is thoroughly mixed. Serve immediately.

Salad with Quinoa and Black Beans

Ingredients:

Cooked quinoa, black beans, bell peppers, cherry tomatoes, red onion, cilantro, lime juice, olive oil, cumin, salt, and pepper are the ingredients.

Preparation:
Cooked quinoa, rinsed black beans, sliced bell peppers, split cherry tomatoes, finely chopped red onion, and chopped cilantro should all be combined in a large mixing dish. To create the dressing, mix together lime juice, olive oil, ground cumin, salt, and pepper in a small bowl. Toss the salad with the dressing until everything is completely covered. Chill before serving.

Chicken Breast Baked with Roasted Vegetables

Ingredients:
Chicken breast, broccoli, cauliflower, carrots, olive oil, garlic powder, paprika, salt, and pepper are the ingredients.

Preparation:
On a baking pan, place the chicken breast. Season with garlic powder, paprika, salt, and pepper and drizzle with olive oil. Toss the broccoli florets, cauliflower florets, and sliced carrots with olive oil, garlic powder, salt, and pepper in a separate dish. Arrange the veggies around the chicken breast on

the same baking sheet. Bake for 20-25 minutes, or until the chicken is well cooked and the veggies are roasted and soft. Serve immediately.

Parfait with Greek Yogurt

Ingredients:
Greek yogurt, berries (strawberries, blueberries, raspberries), granola, and honey (optional).

Preparation:
Layer Greek yogurt, mixed berries, and granola in a glass or dish. If desired, drizzle with honey. Finish with some additional granola and berry sprinkling. Consume as a healthful and filling breakfast or snack.

Salmon Teriyaki with Stir-Fried Vegetables

Ingredients:
Salmon filets, teriyaki sauce, broccoli, snap peas, bell peppers, carrots, garlic, ginger, soy sauce, and sesame oil are the ingredients.

Preparation:

Marinate the salmon filets in the teriyaki sauce for approximately 20 minutes. Heat sesame oil in a skillet or wok over medium heat. Stir in the minced garlic and grated ginger for a minute. Combine the broccoli florets, snap peas, sliced bell peppers, and shredded carrots in a mixing bowl. Cook until the veggies are crisp-tender. Set the veggies aside after removing them from the skillet. Cook the marinated salmon filets in the same skillet over medium heat until they are cooked through and flake easily with a fork. Pour the teriyaki sauce from the marinade into the pan and let it thicken slightly for a minute. Serve the cooked salmon filets with the stir-fried veggies on a platter. Over the fish and veggies, drizzle the teriyaki sauce. Serve immediately.

CHAPTER 8. Salad with Quinoa from the Mediterranean

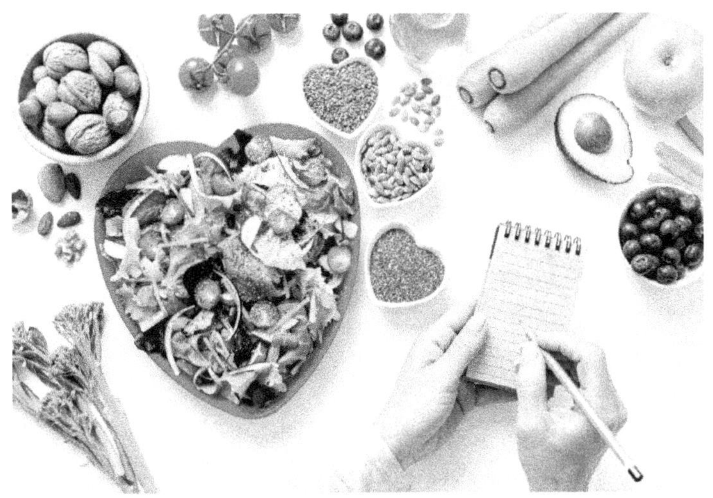

Ingredients:

Cooked quinoa, cherry tomatoes, cucumber, red onion, Kalamata olives, feta cheese, fresh parsley, lemon juice, olive oil, salt, and pepper are the ingredients.

Preparation:

To make the salad, add cooked quinoa, halved cherry tomatoes, diced cucumber, thinly sliced red onion, pitted and split Kalamata olives, crumbled feta cheese, and chopped fresh parsley in a large mixing dish. To create the dressing, mix together lemon juice, olive oil, salt, and pepper in a small bowl. Toss the salad with the dressing until everything is completely covered.

Sweet Potato Bake with Black Bean Salsa

Ingredients:

Sweet potato, black beans, corn, red bell pepper, red onion, cilantro, lime juice, olive oil, cumin, chili powder, salt, and pepper are the ingredients.

Preparation:

Place the sweet potato on a baking sheet and pierce it several times with a fork. Bake the sweet potato for 40-50 minutes, or until soft. To create the salsa, add washed black beans, corn kernels, diced red bell pepper, finely chopped red onion, chopped cilantro, lime juice, olive oil, ground cumin, chili powder, salt, and pepper in a mixing bowl. After the sweet potato is finished cooking, cut it open and ladle the black bean salsa on top. Serve immediately.

Stuffed Bell Peppers with Quinoa

Ingredients:
Bell peppers, cooked quinoa, lean ground turkey or beef, onion, garlic, tomato sauce, Italian seasoning, salt, and pepper are among the ingredients.

Preparation:
Cook ground turkey or beef in a pan until browned. Cook until the chopped onion and minced garlic are softened. Add cooked quinoa, tomato sauce, Italian seasoning, salt, and pepper to taste. Fill the bell peppers with the mixture and lay them on a baking tray. Bake for 25-30 minutes, or until the peppers are soft and the mixture is hot.

Caprese Salad

Ingredients:
Fresh mozzarella cheese, tomatoes, fresh basil leaves, balsamic glaze, olive oil, salt, and pepper are the ingredients.

Preparation:

Prepare the fresh mozzarella cheese and tomatoes by cutting them into rounds. Arrange the slices on a platter in an even pattern, alternating between mozzarella and tomatoes. Between each slice, place a fresh basil leaf. Drizzle with olive oil and balsamic glaze. Season with salt and pepper to taste. As a light and refreshing appetizer or side dish, serve.

Lettuce Wraps with Chicken Fajitas

Ingredients:

Chicken breast, bell peppers, onion, fajita seasoning, lettuce leaves, guacamole, salsa, and sour cream (to taste).

Preparation:

Thinly slice the chicken breast, bell peppers, and onion. Cook the chicken in a pan until it is browned and cooked through. Sprinkle with fajita spice and add the sliced bell peppers and onion. Stir-fry the veggies until they are crisp-tender. Fill lettuce leaves with the chicken and veggie combination. If preferred, top with guacamole, salsa, and a dollop of sour cream. Complete it. Fold the lettuce leaves into wraps and attach with toothpicks if needed. As a tasty and low-carb alternative to typical tortilla wraps, serve the chicken fajita lettuce wraps.

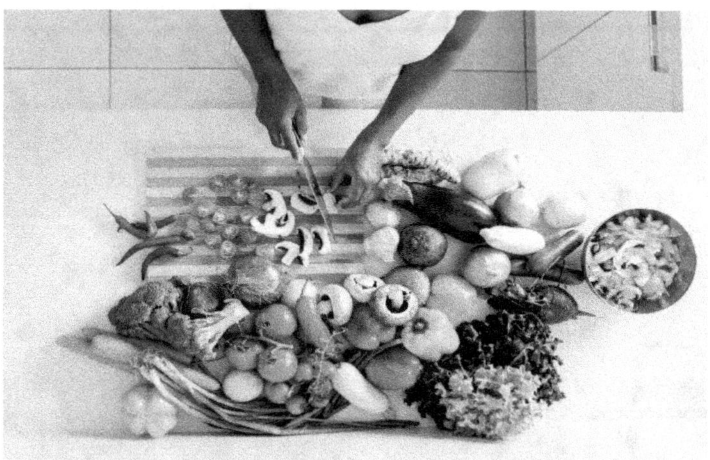

Ingredients:

Spinach leaves, mixed berries (strawberries, blueberries, and raspberries), goat cheese, sliced almonds, and balsamic vinaigrette.

Preparation:

To make the salad, add fresh spinach leaves, mixed berries, crumbled goat cheese, and sliced almonds in a large mixing basin. Toss gently with the balsamic vinaigrette to coat. Serve as a light and healthy salad alternative.

Stir-Fry Tofu with Brown Rice

Ingredients:
Firm tofu, diverse vegetables (broccoli, bell peppers, carrots, and snap peas), garlic, ginger, soy sauce, sesame oil, and brown rice are the main ingredients.

Preparation:
Tofu should be drained and pressed to eliminate extra moisture. Tofu should be cut into cubes. Heat sesame oil in a skillet or wok over medium heat. Stir in the minced garlic and grated ginger for a minute. Stir-fry the tofu cubes until golden brown on both sides. Set the tofu aside after removing it from the pan. Stir-fry the mixed veggies in the same pan until crisp-tender. Return the tofu to the pan and top with soy sauce. Serve the tofu stir-fry with brown rice.

Tzatziki Chicken Skewers from Greece

Ingredients:
Chicken breast, lemon juice, garlic, dried oregano, olive oil, salt, and pepper are the ingredients. Tzatziki sauce is made using Greek yogurt,

cucumber, garlic, fresh dill, lemon juice, salt, and pepper.

Preparation:
Prepare the chicken breast by cutting it into bite-sized pieces. Combine lemon juice, minced garlic, dried oregano, olive oil, salt, and pepper in a mixing bowl. Thread the marinated chicken onto the skewers. Grill the chicken skewers for 8-10 minutes, flipping halfway through, until cooked through. Grate the cucumber and press away the excess liquid for the tzatziki sauce. Combine Greek yogurt, grated cucumber, minced garlic, chopped fresh dill, lemon juice, salt, and pepper in a mixing bowl. To blend, stir everything together well. Serve the grilled chicken skewers beside the tzatziki sauce.

Soup with Quinoa and Vegetables

Ingredients:
Cooked quinoa, vegetable broth, onion, garlic, carrots, celery, bell peppers, zucchini, canned diced tomatoes, dried herbs (such as thyme and oregano), salt, and pepper are just a few of the ingredients.

Preparation:

Sauté diced onion, minced garlic, chopped carrots, chopped celery, diced bell peppers, and sliced zucchini in a large saucepan until slightly softened. Combine canned diced tomatoes, cooked quinoa, dried herbs, vegetable broth, salt, and pepper in a mixing bowl. Allow to simmer for 15-20 minutes, or until the veggies are soft. If necessary, adjust the seasoning. For a filling and healthy supper, serve the quinoa and vegetable soup hot.

In conclusion, "Weight Loss Diet for Beginners" is an excellent resource for anybody starting their weight reduction quest. This book provides readers with the skills they need to reach their weight reduction objectives by giving a thorough guide, practical advice, and scientifically supported solutions. The author's knowledge and sympathetic approach provide a welcoming atmosphere, enabling novices to achieve long-term lifestyle adjustments and establish healthy eating habits. Whether you want to lose a few pounds or entirely improve your health, this book provides a clear path to success. Accept the wisdom contained inside these pages and set out on a transforming path toward a better, happier self.

Furthermore, with a little effort and self-belief, "Weight Loss Diet for Beginners" transforms into a personal coach, leading readers through the ups and downs of their weight reduction journey. The author's encouraging tone and motivational words create confidence in newcomers, reminding them that every step forward, no matter how tiny, puts them closer to their ultimate objectives. With each page flip, readers will be motivated to overcome obstacles, adopt healthy habits, and prioritize their well-being. Remember that success is judged not just by numbers on a scale, but also by the good changes that occur inside. Trust the knowledge of this book, implement its concepts, and observe the amazing outcomes that await you on your weight reduction journey.

APPRECIATION

Dear Valued Customers,

We would like to convey our heartfelt thanks for picking our book and entrusting us with your time. Your steadfast support and useful comments are genuinely valued. As we always endeavor to strengthen our work and produce engaging information, we respectfully seek your support by submitting an honest evaluation. Your evaluations carry tremendous value, not just for us as writers but also for potential readers seeking educated judgments. Whether you found our book amazing or feel there are places that may be improved, we sincerely appreciate your ideas and comments.

Your feedback serves as a continuing source of encouragement for us to develop tales that profoundly connect with you. We humbly urge you to spend a few seconds to leave your review on Amazon, since your comments contain the capacity to substantially affect the success and reach of our book, enabling it to touch a broader audience.

Remember, your review need not be long or extremely complicated. Simply expressing your honest opinions, emphasizing the things that connected with you, or identifying important components would be incredibly beneficial. Once again, we express our deepest thanks for being a part of our journey as writers. Your continuous support and involvement are of crucial significance to us. We anxiously await reading your feedback and developing alongside you.

Best regards!

9 798851 302046